# END

# Grey Hair

## Stop and reverse grey Hair naturally

I0447543

**Nazeem Nour**

## Disclaimer

Although in this book you will only find natural and risk free advices and suggestions, the author of this book is not responsible for any incident that might happen after following the steps. If you suffer from any condition or if you have doubts, please consult a practitioner before following the steps of the program.

# Introduction

One day, on a sunny afternoon i was sitting in a park. And while i was there, i was looking at the grass in front of me. The grass was yellow due to too much sun. I know this park very well because I go there almost every day; this is why I can notice all the changes, even the little ones. That's why I know the grass wasn't like that a week ago, it was green; but because of a sunny week, the heat from the sun "burnt" the grass and gave it this yellow color. A week after that when we had less sunny days, the grass recovered its green color. The same thing happened when it hasn't rained for a long time. Due to lack of water the grass becomes yellowish.

This means that in order for the grass to be green ( it's original color) it needs to be under certain conditions: an appropriate amount of sun , an appropriate amount of water ...It also means that the grass can go from a green color , to yellow and back to green in another way , it can heal !

The reason why I am talking about this ,is because I believe that your hair is like the grass it can go from dark to grey when it's not given what it needs , and then from grey to dark when given it needs. Nature has its ways of giving us lessons.

I know that if you are reading these lines, it's probably because you are having grey hair and you want it to stop. Maybe you are young and you are embarrassed or disturbed because you feel like you are getting older before time .Or maybe you are a little bit old and you want to stay young and take care of your look. For whatever reason you want to stop having grey hair you are in the right place , and this book is going to show you exactly how to stop and reverse grey hair.

Why are you having grey hair?

But before I start showing you what you need to do to get rid of your grey hair, let's discuss why you are having it? The principal reason is that you have a bad life style. Grey hair didn't start appearing suddenly. It came there because of many years of bad habits like bad diet, too much stress... this is often the main cause of grey hair. What you do on a daily basis is very important if you want to stop and reverse grey hair.

Another reason is genetics. Ok I know what you are thinking: it's from your parents or great parents and there is nothing you can do about it? Well you are wrong. By following the steps in this program you can do a lot. And if you stick to the program for a long time you can forget about genetics. Your lifestyle can beat genetics.

Another main reason is what we call chronic stress. Let's imagine that John has a wife that he loves so much, and one god forbid, John lost his wife. John became very sad and spent many days mourning his wife. The stress caused by the loss of his wife and the sadness and all the negative emotions could cause you to have grey hair.

Your hair is connected to your body; this is why we cannot address the problem of grey hair without considering your whole body.

Also you need to be patient, because in this book you won't find a magic formula that will get rid of your grey hair. This program needs discipline. Sure you will start to see results in just few days, if you want longue lasting results you need more than just few days. Stop your grey hair take some time but reversing your hair takes much longer.

So let's start:

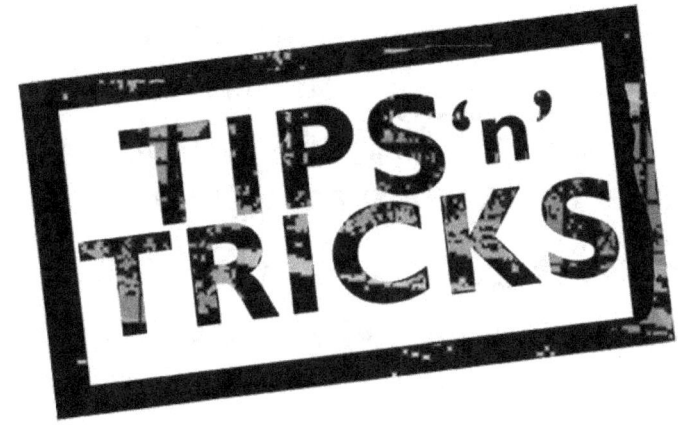

# 1

# Tricks for instant results

When you start having grey hair at an early age and you feel embarrassed, or you want them to disappear, what you can do is cut few grey hair here and there, this way you will reduce the number of grey hair. We the help of a relative or your barber cut the most apparent ones.

You can also choose a haircut that will hide your grey hair. For example cut your hair to a minimum on each side (if you have grey hair on the side around the ear).

Another way is to use a good quality cream or oil for hair. This will make your hair shine, the color of your hair brighter, and hide your grey hair. There are many products out there, feel free to experiment. Be careful not to use a product with a lot of chemicals that might hurt your hair.

This is only a temporary solution and a way to hide your grey instantly without too much effort.

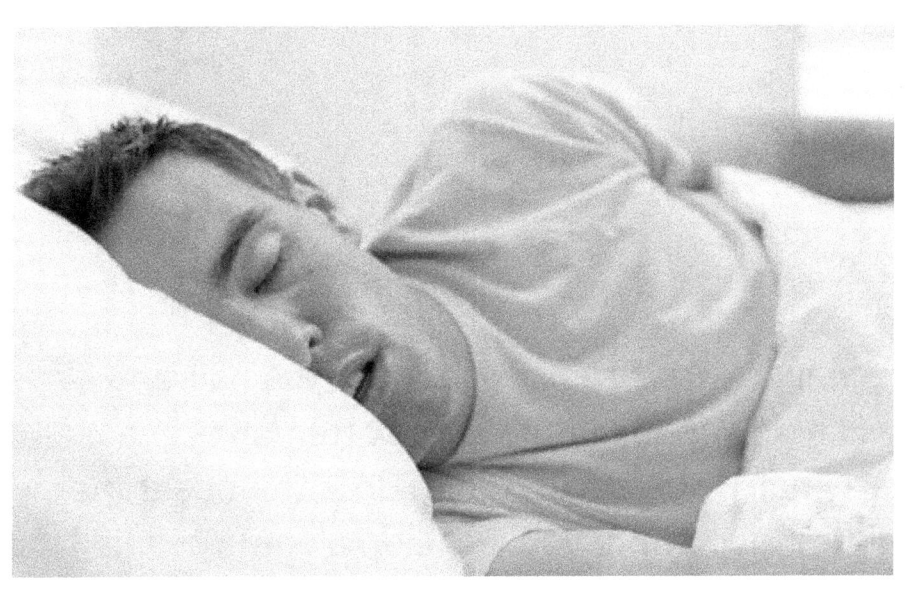

# 2

# Sleep

Sleep a lot: sleeping is good for the hair and it will help you manage stress better (stress causes grey hair). The best thing to do is to not set the alarm, sleep until you wake up alone. You will easily notice that when you don't sleep well your hair (and your skin) doesn't look good. You will notice more grey hair.

So make sure to go to sleep early this way you can get at least eight hours of sleep and more. Don't miss this step very important.

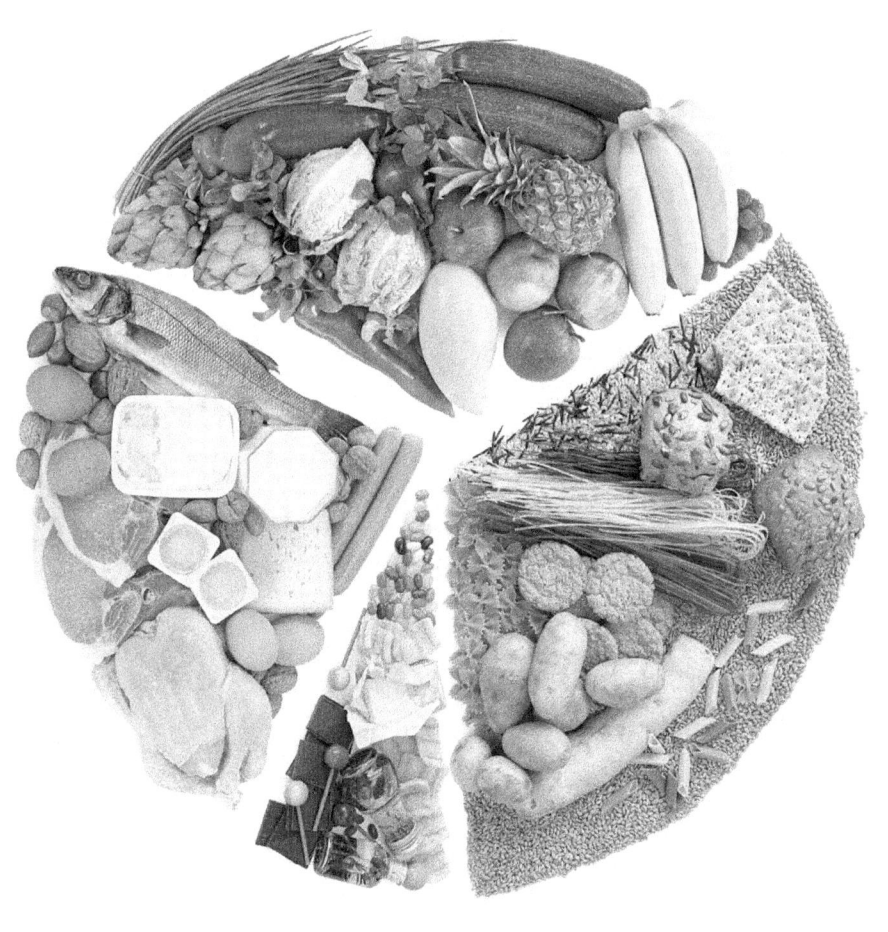

# 3
# Food

Food is very important for keeping your hair dark. You need to take this part very seriously. Here what you need to eat in order to keep your hair dark and reverse grey hair:

_ Good quality food: seek food that is rich in nutrients like organic food or food without too much chemicals. The vitamins and minerals that are in your food will nourish your hair therefore stop and reverse grey hair. Seek also fresh food or food of the season which contain more nutrients. Try also to eat raw food more often! To avoid grey it's important to focus on vegetables and fruits, eat as much as you can

_ Protein: they are essentials to your hair and nails whether it's chicken, meat or fish. I recommend animal protein because i noticed that it's better than vegetal protein (tofu, beans, seitan, eggs ...). Go for a good portion with each meal: between 100g up to 300g.

_Cereals: Cereals are not that important for keeping your hair dark and reversing grey hair, however you need to have some. Go for brown cereals like brown rice, or whole wheat bread which contain more vitamins and minerals.

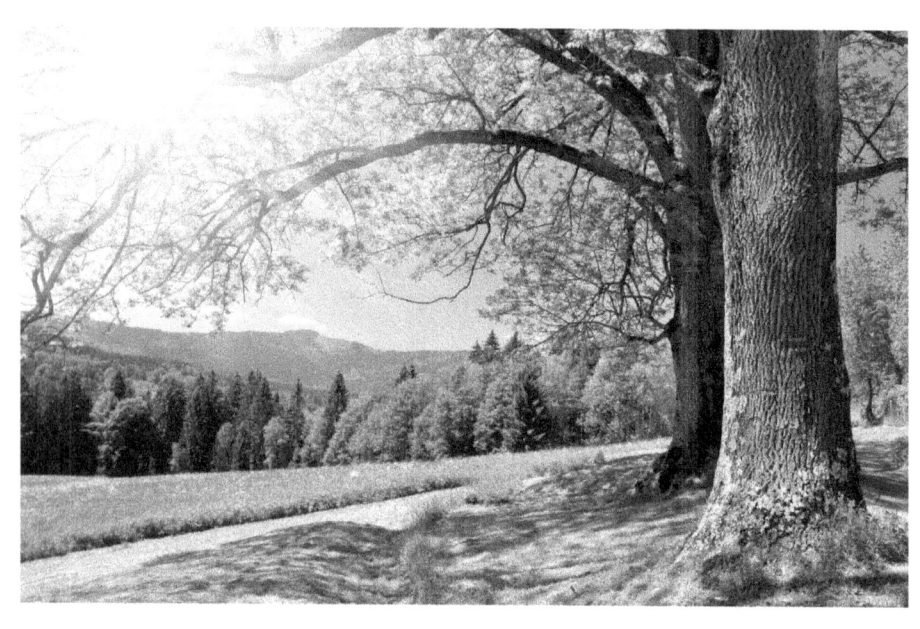

# 4

# Fresh air

Seek fresh air: pollution is not good for your hair and make it grey. Avoid big cities if you can't, go to parks, forest or wherever you can find good quality oxygen...Do this at least 5 days a week for minimum 20 min. the more the better. Good quality air is very important for your hair. Sadly today the air is polluted, combine to that bad food and stress, there you have a recipe for grey hair. Try to spend your holidays in the countryside or on the mountain. You should spend at least one month in a natural environment. Two months is good .Do breathing exercises, any breathing exercise you like?

One exercise that i like in particular: Breathe in from one nostril and hold it as much as you can then breath one from the other nostril. Do the same in the other sens: breathe in from the other nostril (you just exhaled from) hold then breathe out from the other side.

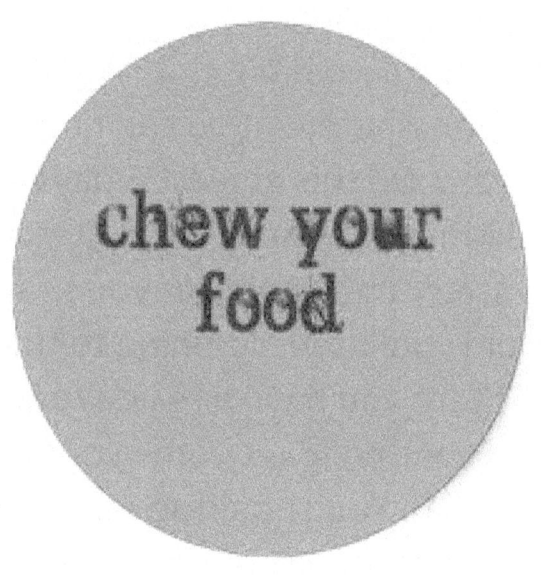

# 5

# Chew

Chew your food: Chew your food hard, this will strengthen the muscle around your teeth and then your head, this will bring more blood to your hair and improve blood circulation. The blood will nourish your hair with the nutrients from the food and keeps it from becoming grey and after a while reversing the color from grey to the original color.

Food is becoming softer and softer (like junk food) seek good food that you can chew hard. When you are chewing your food, hold your teeth clunged together for three to five second, this will reinforce the muscles and bring more blood to your scalp.

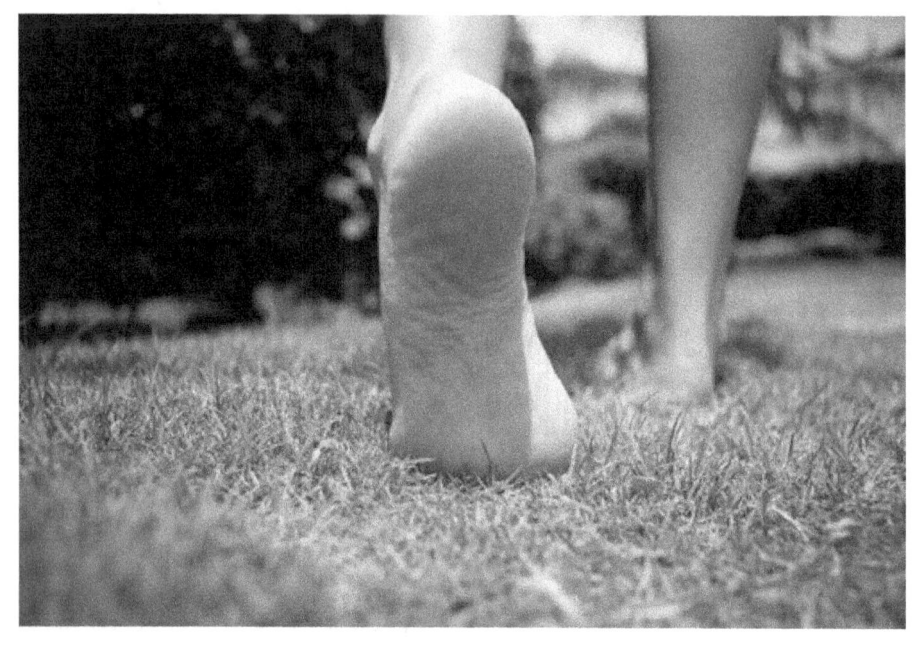

# 6
# Earthing

Earthing: take off your shoes and ground yourself to the earth, it's good for your hair. Do this at least 5 days a week for 20 min. the more the better. Earthing is a new and a natural way to energize your body and your hair. The energy that comes from the earth goes through your body up to your scalp and hair and nourishes it. This way your hair doesn't turn grey.

You will find a lot of information on earthing and it's benefits, if you have never heard of it , i advice you to do some research on it , this way you will have a better idea on what i am talking about .

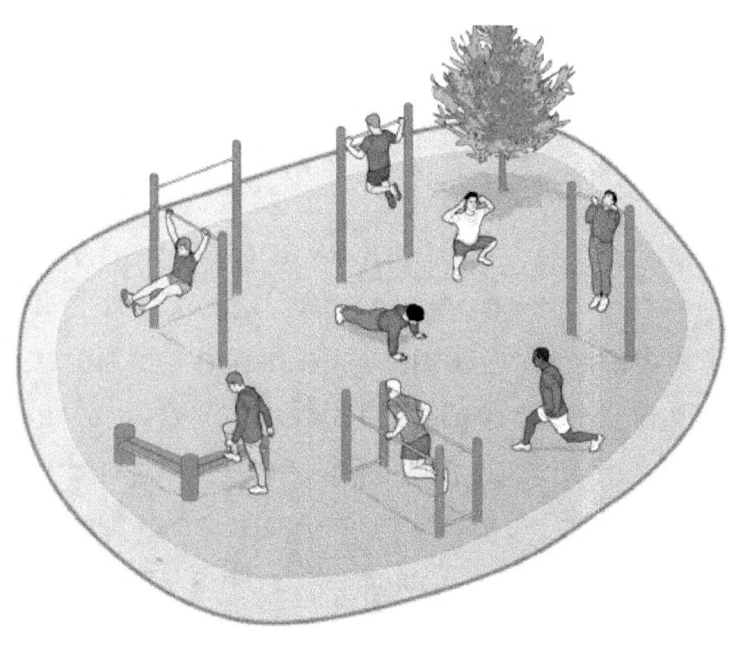

# 7

# Exercise

Combine cardio with lifting/strength.

Exercises like push-ups, burpees, mountain climber ... are good for your hair. The swing of the kettlebell is also good. If you go to the gym focus on three exercises: dead lift, bench press and squat with this three exercises you work out your body and you increase blood circulation in your head and scalp and reverse your grey hair.

The goal is to perform some type of vigorous activity for a minimum of 15 to 30 minutes, three to five times a week. This vigorous activity should be executed in between 60% to 80% of your Maximum Heart Rate (MHR)

How to calculate your MHR:

*a) - subtract your current age from 220. This number is your MHR.*

*b) - Multiply this number by 0.60. This is 60 percent of your MHR.*

*C) - take the number you came up with in step a). Multiply it by 0.80. This is 80 percent of your MHR.*

These numbers of 60 percent and 80 percent represent the range of your Target Heart Rate (THR). (An important note: many high blood pressure medications work by lowering the heart rate, which would mean that your MHR and target rates may need to be lowered as well. If you are taking any blood pressure medications, contact your physician to find out how best to adjust these numbers. )

When engaging in exercise, you will need to keep track of your heart rate to make sure you are staying within the 60 percent to 80 percent THR range. This is commonly done by lightly pressing the index finger of the right hand over the artery just under the skin on the skin on the inside of the left wrist. The rate is easily determined by counting the beats for 15 seconds, the multiplying that number by 4. This will be your heart rate. (Or count the beats for one minute)

If you don't like this way of counting your heart beats, there is an alternative rule of thumb: if you can hold a conversation, you aren't working hard enough. If you can sing, you are not working hard enough either. If you are out of breath, or have to stop and catch your breath, you're definitely working too hard. Stay in between!

Also it's important that you find an activity that you enjoy. There are a lot of activities out there, so find something that you enjoy. The main point here is to get your circulation going.

Exercise outside for maximum oxygen intake which will stimulate your scalp. But don't forget that chewing your food hard is the best exercise for hair loss.

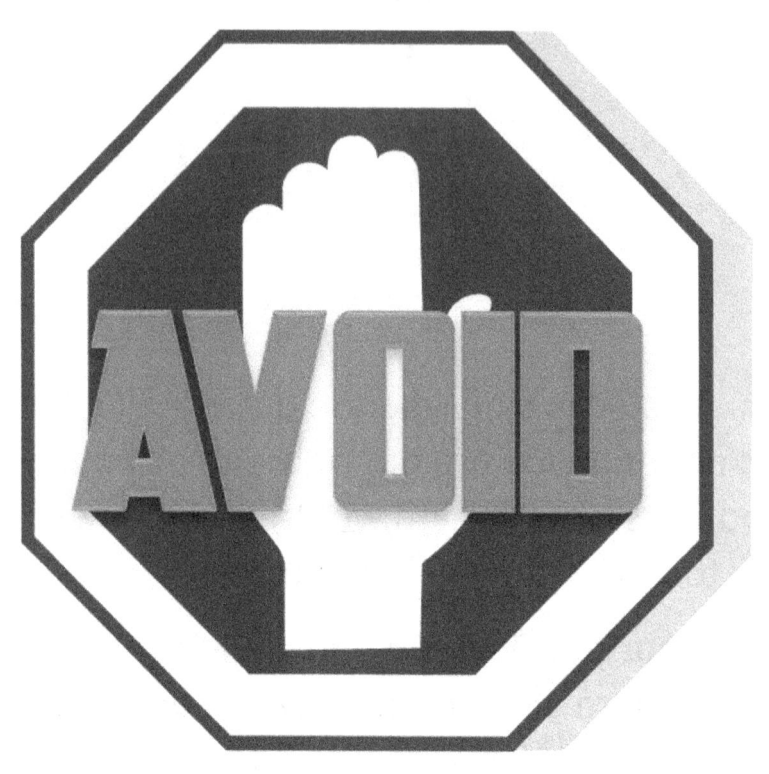

8

# What to avoid

What to avoid: Sugar, coffee

_ Sugar: Brian Tracy calls it a poison. Sugar is not only bad for your body and your health but it is also bad for your hair. The less you eat it the better.

_ Coffee: For the sake of the color your hair choose tea over coffee. Drinking coffee once or twice a day for years could turn your hair grey.

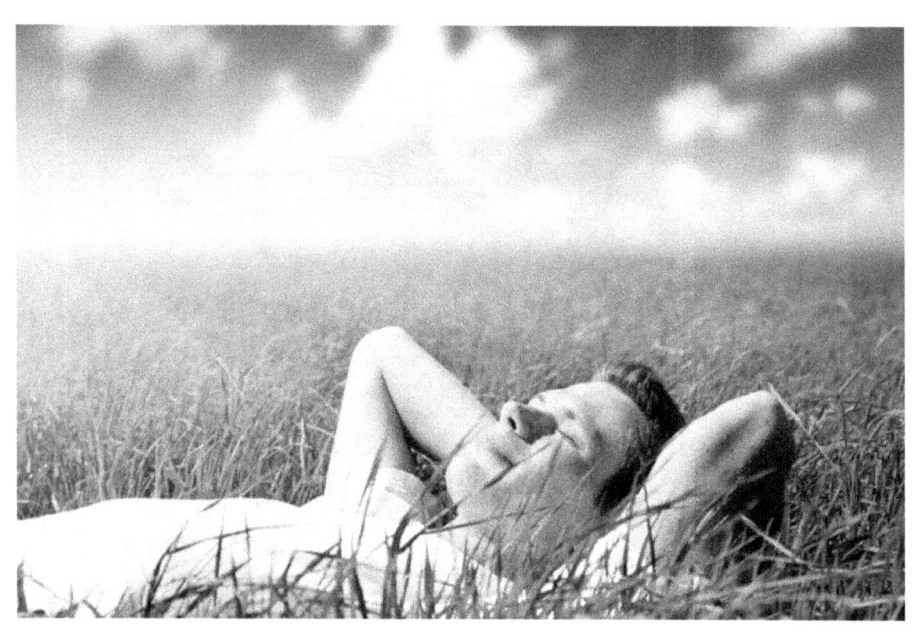

# 9

# Relax and Rest

Rest: learn to rest during the day. Take a nap or a hot bath... Take breaks to avoid stress. Resting is important and it allows you to conserve physical energy.

I personally noticed that that the color of my hair is better on my days off than on my working days. So if you care about your hair, conserve your energy. You might need to think of a way to work less and earn more, there are many solutions out there that will show you how to do it. Check out the book of Tim Ferriss *"The Four Hour Workweek"* for a start.

Work on your thought, think positive, meditate, focus on the present, do things that make you feel good, listen to relaxing music.... Worrying stresses you and makes your hair turn grey. Everyday do an activity that calms you and relaxes you: take a walk; a bath; meditate even for 5 minutes ...

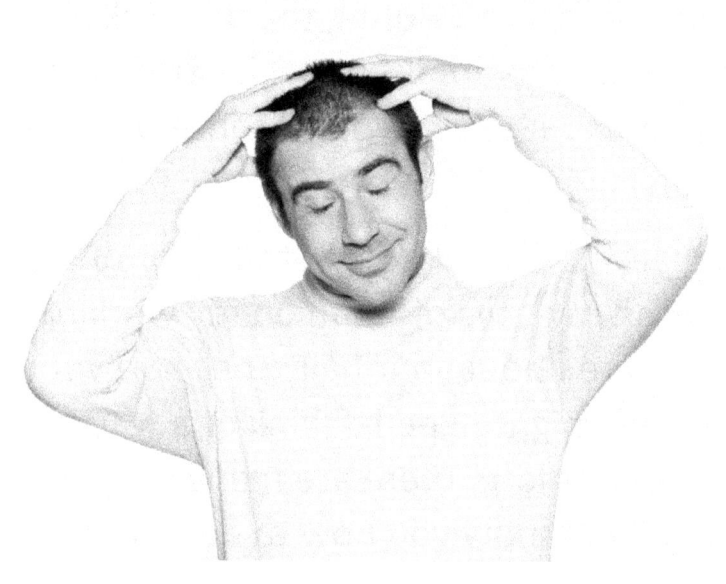

# 10

# Massage

Massage your scalp: massaging will bring more blood to your scalp and nourish your hair. There are many exercises out there you can do any massaging exercise you want. The most important rule to follow is: don't use your nails when massaging. Your nails might hurt your hair.

Here are some exercises:

_ Hanging: Lay on your back on a bed or table hang your head off the edge so that blood circulation is increased through the neck and scalp. Breathe deeply and relax. Lie there for several minutes

_ Forehead Manipulation: Hold your left hand across the back of your head to steady your neck relaxes your head into your hand. Place your right hand across your forehead, stretching your thumb and forefinger across your brow line. Move your hand slowly and firmly upward to one inch past your hairline. Repeat four or five times.

_ Scalp manipulation: Place the palms of your hands firmly against your scalp above each ear. «Lift" the scalp in a circular movement, first with the hands at the side of your head, then with one hand at the top front and the other at the center back, right at the nape of your neck.

_Hairline Circles: Beginning at the hairline, place this fingers of both hands on the center of your hair line - right at your forehead. Massage around the hairline, concentrating on the areas of hair loss as you work your fingertips in a gentle circular motion. Work all the way around your hairline, including the temples, behind your ears, across the back of your neck.

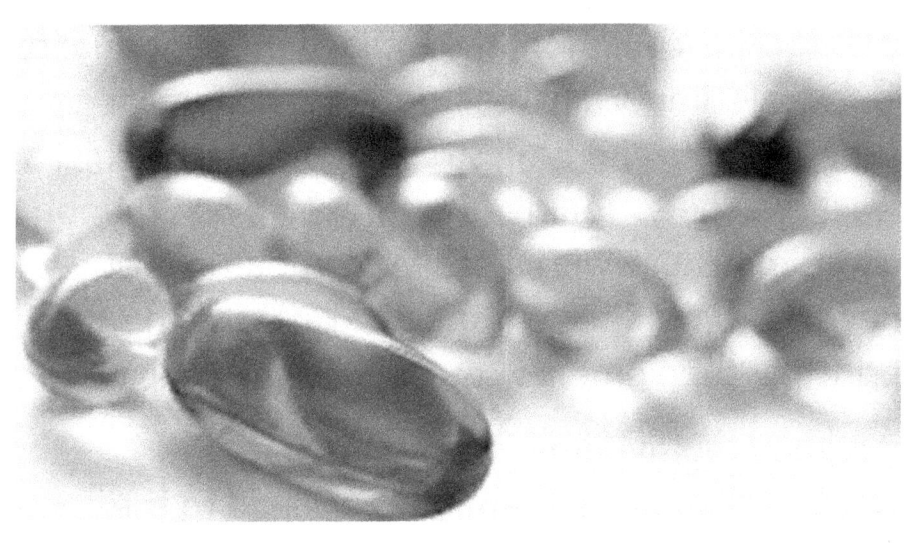

# 11

# Take Supplements

Adding high-quality supplements can help you maintain the natural color of your hair and reverse the grey hair. Keep in the forefront of your mind that for this condition, the topic of nutrient quality is critically important, as for the food. Regular supermarkets and drug stores do not carry a high level of quality. You need to shop at a health food or vitamin store with a positive reputation. Don't hesitate to try different brands. Here are the three principal supplements you need to take daily:

_ A good multivitamin and multimineral combination supplement. This will add to the vitamins and minerals from the food you eat.

_Add a full symphony antioxidant mix once each day. One pill might include: zinc, selenium, N-acetylcysteine, grape seed extract and so forth. Antioxidants are very important for keeping you young.

_ Include an ample dose of omega-3 fatty acids. A dose of 500mg daily is good.

_ add some amino acid mix. 1 gram daily is good.

# How to apply all this

There you have all the steps that you need to follow in order to stop and reverse your grey hair. It will take some times, I won't lie to you: maybe a few days, few weeks or one, two, three months to see results. But on the bright side not only your hair will benefit from following this program, but your health in general will improve.

Here what I advise you to do: take 90 days to work on all the steps each day, focus on this program for this period of time, and dedicate yourself. At the end of the three months you will notice that your grey hair disappeared and that you look much younger.

So good luck!

www.ingramcontent.com/pod-product-compliance
Lightning Source LLC
Chambersburg PA
CBHW070246290526
45789CB00004B/1789